Neuromuscular Medicine: An Outline of High-yield Topics

Michael S. Cartwright, MD, MS

Professor of Neurology
Wake Forest School of Medicine
Winston-Salem, North Carolina, USA

Copyright © 2020 Michael S. Cartwright

All rights reserved.

ISBN-13: 9798645936723

To Sarah, Adam, Alex, and Emma.

CONTENTS

Introduction — Page i

Chapter 1: Muscle — Page 1

Chapter 2: Junction — Page 14

Chapter 3: Nerve — Page 17

Chapter 4: General Neuromuscular Topics — Page 26

Chapter 5: Clinical Neurophysiology — Page 29

Introduction

This text is organized in an extended outline format with many charts and lists, and it is intended to serve as a high-yield study guide for physicians taking board examinations. This text will also serve as a quick clinical guide for all physicians involved in the care of patients with neuromuscular conditions, though it is important to remember that many aspects of neuromuscular medicine are rapidly changing.

A "distal-to-proximal" organizational approach is used, with muscle, then neuromuscular junction, and then nerve discussed as the first three chapters. Within each of these chapters there are brief outlines of normal function, biopsy findings (if applicable), inherited diseases, acquired diseases, and other considerations. Chapter 4 then encompasses general neuromuscular topics, and Chapter 5 includes high-yield electrophysiology concepts. Purposeful redundancy is included to help reinforce topics.

Chapter 1. MUSCLE

Muscle Fiber Types

Type 1   slow twitch, fatigue resistant, lots of mitochondria
Type 2a   moderately fast twitch, fatigue resistant
Type 2x   fast twitch, fatigue resistant
Type 2b   very fast twitch, fatigable
Type 2c   common in fetal and regenerating muscle

The majority of muscle fibers are <u>extrafusal</u>. These are innervated by alpha motor neurons, and the combination of an alpha motor neuron and the extrafusal muscle fibers it innervates is the motor unit. <u>Intrafusal</u> muscle fibers are rare, buried in muscle, and contain stretch receptors that participate in the reflex arc.

The <u>sarcomere</u> (between two Z disks) is the contractile complex of muscle and includes actin (the thin filament with 3 components: actin, tropomyosin, and troponin) and myosin (the thick filament with a single tail and two heads; acts as an ATPase and cross-bridge). Aspects of the sarcomere include:
> H Zone – Thick filaments only
> I Band – Thin filaments only
> A Band – Thick and thin filaments

Muscle Biopsy

ATPase stains can be conducted at 3 different pHs:
> 4.3   Type 1 fibers are dark, Type 2 fibers are light
> 4.6   Type 1 fibers are dark, Type 2a fibers are light, Type 2b fibers are in-between
> 9.4   Type 1 fibers are light, Type 2 fibers are dark

There are other stains used to reveal specific conditions:
> Congo red – individuals with amyloidosis will have apple green birefringence on polarized light and red with rhodamine optics
> Gomori trichrome – highlights ragged-red fibers and nemaline rods
> Succinate dehydrogenase (SDH) – highlights ragged-blue fibers
> Electron microscopy – reveals nemaline rods, inclusion body neurofilaments, paracrystaline inclusions with mitochondria, myosin loss with critical illness myopathy

Neurogenic biopsy findings in muscles include: group atrophy, target fibers (from reinnervation), angular atrophy, and fiber type grouping (from reinnervation). If one muscle fiber of a specific type is completely surrounded by the same type of muscle fibers, this is considered <u>fiber type grouping.</u>

Myopathic biopsy findings in muscles include: internal nuclei, rounded atrophy, and fiber splitting. Muscular dystrophies have necrotic muscle fibers and replacement of muscle fibers with fat and connective tissue (these are considered chronic changes).

Dystrophic myopathy – necrotic muscle fibers, replacement of muscle fibers with fat and connective tissue.

Necrotizing myopathy – causes of this condition include autoimmune, paraneoplastic, "overlap" (connective tissue disease), and toxic (medications, such as statins). A biopsy will demonstrate necrotic muscle fibers with minimal inflammation.

Inclusion body myositis (IBM) – the biopsy will show rimmed vacuoles, endomysial inflammation with CD8+ T cells, invasion of non-necrotic fibers.

Dermatomyositis (DM) vs polymyositis (PM) – DM with perivascular and perifascicular inflammation (closer to the skin) with CD4+ cells, PM with endomysial inflammation with CD8+ cells.

Mitochondrial Myopathy – ragged-red fibers (Gomori), ragged-blue fibers (SDH), cox negative fibers.

McArdle disease – no myophosphorylase staining in type 2 fibers.

Critical illness myopathy – loss of myosin and breakdown of sarcomeres, which is demonstrated well with electron microscopy.

Spinal muscular atrophy (SMA) – this is a motor neuron disease, so there will be a neurogenic pattern of prominent fiber type grouping, angular atrophy, and some enlarged fibers.

Inherited Myopathies

Congenital Myopathies (congenital onset, relatively static; rods, cores, and central nuclei are often present; no dystrophic findings on biopsy)

Myopathy	Chromosome/Gene/Protein	Unique Finding(s)
Nemaline rod myopathy	5 different genes (*ACTA1*, beta tropomyosin, troponin t1, nebulin, cofilin-2)	-Rods on Gomori trichrome -Variable presentation -Can be infantile and severe -Late-onset form occurs with proximal weakness and head drop, even into adulthood -High palate
Central core disease	-Autosomal dominant (AD) -*RYR* Ryanodine gene	-Malignant hyperthermia -Type 1 fibers with cores
Multiminicore	*SEPN1* Selenoprotein gene	
Myotubular (centronuclear) myopathy	-*MTM1* (myotubularin, x-linked) gene -*DMN2* (dynamin, AD) gene	-Ophthalmoplegia -Head is narrow and elongated -Respiratory involvement -Decrement on rep stim -Biopsy: central nuclei with halo around them, spokes radially from nuclei looks like a necklace

Congenital Muscular Dystrophies (congenital onset, autosomal recessive (AR), contractures common, some are static and some progress, secondary to a problem with extracellular matrix binding to muscle fibers, dystrophic biopsy findings, can be split into <u>merosin negative and positive</u> or <u>syndromic and non-syndromic</u>)

Myopathy	Chromosome/Gene/Protein	Unique Finding(s)
Laminin a2 (merosin) deficiency	*MDCD* gene	-Non-syndromic -50% of all congenital muscular dystrophies
Bethlem (less severe)/Ullrich (more severe)	Collagen (*COL6A*) gene	Non-syndromic
Walker-Warburg	*POMT1/2* genes	Syndromic
Fukuyama	*FKTN* gene, fukutin protein	-Syndromic -Seizures -Low IQ
Muscle-eye-brain Muscular dystrophy-dystroglycanopathies		-Syndromic -Seizures -Low IQ

Muscular Dystrophies (onset in childhood or as an adult, dysfunction of cell-membrane complex, progressive, dystrophic biopsy findings, limb-girdle muscular dystrophy categorization changed in 2017)

Myopathy	Chromosome/Gene/Protein	Unique Finding(s)
Duchenne/Becker Dystrophinopathies	-X-linked -Duchenne: 65% with large exon deletions, 35% point mutation, 5% duplication; out-of-frame mutations result in no dystrophin production -Becker's with in-frame mutations maintaining some dystrophin production	-Calf pseudohypertrophy -Cardiomyopathy -Mother with cardiomyopathy -Treat with oral steroids once motor milestones plateau -20% can be treated with IV eteplirsen or golodirsen anti-sense oligonucleotides
Facioscapulohumeral (FSHD)	-AD -Chromosome 4, two genes involved: *D4Z4* trinucleotide deletion & *DUX4* toxic gain-of-function	-Scapular winging -Facial weakness -Asymmetric -Variable penetrance -Often have myalgias
Oculopharyngeal (OPMD)	-AD -GCG trinucleotide repeat - *PABPN1/2* gene	-Ptosis -Ophthalmoparesis -Dysphagia
Emery-Dreifuss	-*LMNA* gene -Emerin gene -*SYNE* genes	-Contractures -Cardiac conduction abnormalities -Nuclear proteins

Limb-girdle Muscular Dystrophies (onset in childhood or as an adult, dysfunction of cell-membrane complex, progressive, dystrophic biopsy findings, limb-girdle muscular dystrophy categorization changed in 2017)

Limb-girdle Dominant (LGMDD) (used to be Type 1)	LGMDs are listed in the order in which they were discovered	-AD -Less severe -Less common
LGMDD 4	Myotilin	
LGMDD 5	*COL6A*	-Bethlem -Contractures
LGMD Recessive (LGMDR) (used to be called Type 2)	LGMDs are listed in the order in which they were discovered	-AR -More severe -More common
LGMDR 1	Calpain	-Posterior thigh and pelvis -Contractures of calf/elbow -Common in Spain and South Europe -High CK -No cardiac involvement -Symmetric scapular winging -Similar presentation to FSHD
LGMDR 2	Dysferlin, allelic with Miyoshi myopathy	-Also causes distal myopathy involving the gastrocnemius -High CK
LGMDR 3-6	Sarcoglycanopathies	
LGMDR 8	*TRIM* gene	
LGMDR 9	*FKRP* gene, fukutin	-Dilated cardiomyopathy -Common in North Europe
LGMDR 12	*ANO5* gene	-Common -Proximal leg weakness

Distal Myopathies (rimmed vacuoles, usually no facial involvement – except myotonic dystrophy)

Myopathy	Chromosome/Gene/Protein	Unique Finding(s)
Myotonic dystrophy 1		-Common -See under "dystrophic myotonias"
Miyoshi (dysferlin)	AR, chromosome 2, allelic with LGMDR 2	-No rimmed vacuoles -High CK -Medial gastrocnemius affected
Myofibrillar (desmin) myopathy	AD, multiple genes (filamin, myotilin, bag-3, z-band)	-Can be distal and/or proximal weakness -Cardiomyopathy -Neuropathy -Fibs and positive waves on EMG -Muscle biopsy pattern -Z disk disorder -Congo-red abnormalities -NADH with abnormal vacuoles -Desmin aggregates
Laing distal myopathy	AD, Myosin heavy chain 7 (*MYH7*)	-Presents in teens -Foot drop -Cardiomyopathy
Welander distal myopathy	AD	-Later life (30-40s) -Starts in upper limb with extensor/flexor weakness
Udd distal myopathy	AD, titin gene on chromosome 2	-Later life (30-50s) -Causes foot drop
Nonaka		-Onset in 20s -Foot drop -Rimmed vacuoles

Dystrophic Myotonias

Myopathy	Chromosome/Gene/Protein	Unique Findings
Myotonic dystrophy 1 (DM1) Steinert	AD, chromosome 19, *DMPK* gene, CTG repeat	-Cataracts -90% have cardiac conduction abnormalities -Endocrinopathies -Congenital with > 1000 repeats
Myotonic dystrophy 2 (DM2) Proximal myotonic myopathy (PROMM)	AD, chromosome 3, zinc finger 9 gene, CCTG repeat	Proximal
Schwartz-Jampel Chondrodystrophic myotonia		Short stature

Non-dystrophic Myotonias (no cardiac problems)

Myopathy	Chromosome/Gene/Protein	Unique Findings
Myotonia congenita	*CLCN1* chloride channel Chromosome 7	-Muscle hypertrophy -Better with activity -No effect of cooling -Dominant (Thomsen) -Recessive (Becker) -After discharges with compound muscle action potential (CMAP) -Short exercise with electrical decrement that then resolves
Paramyotonia congenita	-*CLCN1* chloride channel and -*SCN4* sodium channel Chromosome 7 and 17	-Worse with activity and cooling -Cooling increases discharges -After discharges with CMAP -Short exercise with electrical decrement that then worsens
Hyperkalemic periodic paralysis (hyperKPP)	*SCN4* sodium channel Chromosome 17	-AD -Worse with activity -Frequent, mild PP attacks -Similar to phenotype to paramyotonia congenita

Periodic Paralyses (absent reflexes, bulbar and respiratory muscles spared, thyroid conditions can mimic these)

Myopathy	Chromosome/Gene/Protein	Unique Findings
HypoKPP	-AD -Type 1 - *CACNA1S* Calcium channel -Type 2 - SCN4 Sodium channel	-Severe attacks -Triggered by large carbohydrate meal -Can develop fixed myopathy later in life
HyperKPP	*SCN4* Sodium channel	-Like paramyotonia -Myotonic discharges on EMG
Anderson-Tawil	*KCNJ2* Potassium channel	-Periodic paralysis -Hypertelorism -Prolonged QT
Gitelman Syndrome	*SLC12A3*	-Loss of multiple electrolytes from kidney -Results in hypokalemia
Brody disease	*ATP2A1* (SERCA calcium channel)	-Stiffness -Difficulty relaxing muscles

Metabolic Myopathies - Glycogen/glucose or lipid storage disorders. Similar clinical presentation to mitochondrial myopathies.

Glycogen storage diseases ((GSD) vacuolar myopathy with periodic acid-Schiff positive material, most have AR inheritance, worse with brief and intense exercise)

Myopathy	Chromosome/Gene/Protein	Unique Findings
GSD II (Pompe, acid alpha-glucosidase deficiency (GAA), acid maltase deficiency)	*GAA* gene	-Biopsy with punctate acid phosphatase positivity -Lysosomal -LGMD presentation -Lumbar paraspinal myotonia -Respiratory involvement -Check GAA on dried blood -Enzyme replacement therapy available (alglucosidase alpha)
GSD IIb (Danon disease, *LAMP-2* gene mutation)	X-linked	-Cognitive delay -Cardiomyopathy -Early-onset proximal weakness
GSD III (Cori or Forbes)		-Debranching enzyme deficiency -Short stature -Hepatomegaly
GSD V (McArdle, myophosphorylase deficiency)	Mutation in *PYGM* gene	-CK remains elevated between episodes of myoglobinuria -Second wind phenomenon -Muscles swell -Benefits from carbohydrate rich diet
GSD VII (Tauri, phosphofructokinase deficiency)		Elevated bilirubin
Debrancher enzyme deficiency		-Hepatomegaly -Cardiomyopathy

Lipid storage disease (worse with long exercise, fasting, and cold temperature)

Myopathy	Chromosome/Gene/Protein	Unique Findings
Carnitine palmitoyltransferase (CPT) II deficiency	*CPT2* gene	-Most frequent cause of recurrent myoglobinuria -Elevation of long-chain acylcarnitine fraction (disease of long-chain fatty acids) -Decreased CPT II enzyme level on muscle biopsy -Muscle biopsy is normal in between attacks -No second-wind phenomenon -Treat with bezafibrate
Co-Q10 deficiency		Elevation of all length fatty acids

Mitochondrial Myopathies (short stature, hearing loss, ocular involvement, ragged-red fibers on Gomori trichrome stain and ragged-blue fibers on SDH stain, cox-negative fibers)

Inheritance patterns:
  Mitochondrial DNA (mtDNA) – from mother to all offspring, spontaneous defects are more likely to occur
  Nuclear DNA – inherited through typical Mendelian patterns, but affects mitochondria

Myopathy	Chromosome/Gene/Protein	Unique Findings
Progressive external ophthalmoplegia (PEO)	Twinkle gene	Ophthalmoplegia
Kearns-Sayre	Most often spontaneous mutation, large mtDNA deletion	-Ophthalmoplegia -Retinopathy -Cardiac conduction abnormalities
Myoclonic epilepsy and ragged red fibers (MERRF)	mtDNA mutations	-Myoclonic epilepsy -Neck lipomas
Mitochondrial encephalopathy, lactic acidosis, and stroke-like episode (MELAS)	mtDNA mutations	Stroke-like syndrome
* Neuropathy, ataxia, and retinitis pigmentosa (NARP)		-Neuropathy -Retinitis pigmentosa
* Mitochondrial neurogastrointestinal encephalopathy syndrome (MNGIE)	AR	-Demyelinating neuropathy -GI symptoms -Diagnosed by elevated thymidine phosphorylase -White matter changes -No cognitive changes -PEO
* POLG1 (polymerase gamma)	AD or AR	-Nuclear mutation results in multiple mitochondrial DNA deletions -Multisystem involvement: eye, ataxia -Sensory ataxic neuropathy, dysarthria, and ophthalmoparesis (SANDO) syndrome

* Predominantly neuropathies; all others myopathies

Forearm Exercise Test – used when metabolic myopathy suspected, use with caution as it can cause rhabdomyolysis.

Normal – ammonia and lactate double
Poor quality study – neither rise
Glycolytic defect – ammonia rises and lactate does not
Myoadenylate deaminase deficiency (MADD) – ammonia does not rise and lactate does
CPT II – exaggerated rise in ammonia and normal rise of lactate
Mitochondrial – normal rise in ammonia and exaggerated rise of lactate (elevated at baseline)

Immune Mediated Myopathies

Pathology can show inflammation (myositis) or a necrotizing myopathy.

Disease	Features
Polymyositis	-3% paraneoplastic -Endomysial inflammation -CD8+ cells
Dermatomyositis	-50% paraneoplastic -Perifascicular atrophy and inflammation -Perivascular inflammation -CD4+ cells
Inclusion body myositis	-Forearm flexor weakness -Chronic and slowly progressive -Can have neuropathic findings on biopsy and EMG -Cytosolic 5'-nucleotidase 1A antibody (anti-CN-1A)
Necrotizing myopathy	-Rare inflammation -Can be paraneoplastic, autoimmune, or toxic (such as statin-related) -Anti-synthetase antibody -Jo-1 antibody -Signal recognition particle (SRP) antibody – acute or chronic
Overlap myositis	Can be seen in systemic lupus erythematosus, scleroderma, Sjogren's
Paraneoplastic	Test: routine cancer screening plus CA 125, CA 19-9, CT chest/abdomen/pelvis, testicular or transvaginal ultrasound

Infectious myositis

CK may be extremely elevated. Can be viral or bacterial (staph and strep).

Trichinosis

Caused by eating undercooked pork. Symptoms include myalgias, elevated CK, fever, and rash.

Chapter 2. NEUROMUSCULAR JUNCTION

Each nicotinic acetylcholine receptor has 2 binding sites on the alpha subunit. The receptor is closely associated with other transmembrane proteins, including MuSK, LRP4, agrin, Dok7, and rapsyn.

Inherited Myasthenic Syndromes

Congenital Myasthenia Syndromes (mainly AR inheritance, except slow-channel; all respond to pyridostigmine, except acetylcholinesterase deficiency; table organized from presynaptic → synaptic → postsynaptic)

Syndrome	Chromosome/Gene/Protein	Features
Choline acetyltransferase syndrome	*CHAT* gene	-Pre-synaptic -Severe, episodic apnea (aka congenital myasthenia gravis (MG) with episodic apnea) -Treated with pyridostigmine
Acetylcholinesterase deficiency		-Synaptic -Repetitive CMAP -Sluggish pupillary light response -Pyridostigmine worsens it -Wheelchair bound
Slow-channel syndrome	AD, chromosome 2 or 17 AchRec subunit mutation	-Post-synaptic -Repetitive CMAP -Variable presentation -Most progressive -Wrist/finger extensor weakness -Treated with quinidine or fluoxetine
Acetylcholine receptor deficiency		-Post-synaptic
Rapsyn		-Post-synaptic -Can be mistaken for seronegative MG -Facial weakness
Plectin		-Post-synaptic
Dok-7		-Post-synaptic -Eye movement spared -Progressive course -Treated with albuterol

NEUROMUSCULAR MEDICINE: AN OUTLINE OF HIGH-YIELD TOPICS

Autoimmune Myasthenia Gravis

80% AchRec antibody positive – can be ocular, bulbar, or generalized. Worsens 7-10 days after starting prednisone.
10% MuSK positive – young African American females (> 80% female) with bulbar onset, head drop, worsen with acetylcholinesterase inhibitors (may develop fasciculations), and responds to plasmapheresis and rituximab.
10% Seronegative – clinically similar to first group; in this group 3-50% have anti LRP antibodies.

All individuals with autoimmune MG need a CT of the chest to evaluate for thymic hyperplasia. If they have thymic hyperplasia, this necessitates thymectomy. Thymus biopsy almost always shows hyperplasia, but malignancy is possible.

Treatment with acetylcholinesterase inhibitors, thymectomy (generalized disease, age < 65), and/or long-term immunosuppression/immunomodulation (this is the mainstay of treatment). Immunosuppression may include:
- Prednisone
- Azathioprine
- Mycophenolate mofetil
- Methotrexate
- Eculizumab - the only FDA approved treatment; C5 complement antibody; main risk is Neisseria meningitis (encapsulated organism)
- IVIG
- Plasmapheresis.

Myasthenic crisis is treated with IVIG or plasmapheresis. Plasmapheresis may be more efficacious.

Lambert-Eaton Myasthenic Syndrome (LEMS)

P/Q voltage-gated calcium channel antibody, autonomic symptoms (dry mouth), no patellar reflexes, improves with exercise, 50% associated with cancer (usually small cell lung cancer), and these antibodies can also cause cerebellar degeneration. Repetitive stimulation at 2-3 Hz shows a decrement, and at 50 Hz shows an increment. 10 seconds of exercise also produce an increment.

Botulinum Toxin

Patients have dilated pupils and dry mouth, which is different from myasthenia gravis. Should see decrement with 2-3 Hz repetitive stimulation and increment with exercise or 50 Hz repetitive stimulation, similar to LEMS. Can also use mouse bioassay to diagnose.

Types A and B are common, if types C, D, E, F, or G are seen, suspect bioterrorism.

Suspect aerosolized bioterrorism if all individuals in one geographical location are affected and no common food source.

Infantile botulism causes poor suck, hypotonia, and constipation. 50 Hz rep stim shows facilitation/increment. Treatment with botulism immune globulin intravenous (human) is effective.

SNARE proteins mediate fusion of vesicle and pre-synaptic membrane. Botulinum toxin cleaves SNARE proteins and permanently halts acetylcholine release:
- Synaptobrevin or VAMP on vesicle membrane – Botox B on vesicle membrane
- SNAP-25 and syntaxin on the presynaptic membrane – Botox A cleaves SNAP-25 and Botox C cleaves syntaxin

Chapter 3. NERVE

Nerve Types

Motor
        Alpha – motor neuron, fast conducting
        Gamma – intrafusal (contain stretch receptors), medium speed

Sensory
        Type 1a (A alpha) – muscle spindle, fast
        Type 1b (A alpha) – Golgi tendon organ, fast
        Type 2 (A beta)
        Type 3 (A delta) – free nerve endings, fast pain, medium speed, thinly myelinated
        Type 4 (C) – slow pain, slow, no myelin

Autonomic
        Preganglionic (B) – release acetylcholine
        Postganglionic (C) – slow, no myelin

Nerve Biopsy

Infrequently conducted. Usually for suspected vasculitis or amyloidosis.
Teased fiber preparation used for chronic inflammatory demyelinating polyneuropathy (CIDP) (to show demyelination) and hereditary neuropathy with predisposition to pressure palsies (HNPP) (to show tomaculae).
Onion bulbs from demyelination and remyelination in CMT and sometimes CIDP.

Inherited Neuropathies

Charcot-Marie-Tooth (hereditary sensorimotor polyneuropathy)

CMT Type	Chromosome/Gene/Protein	Unique Finding(s)
CMT type 1 (3 and 4 - AR)		-Demyelinating -AD
CMT 1a	Chromosome 17, *PMP22* duplication	-Most common type -Onion bulb formation
CMT 1b	Chromosome 1, *MPZ* gene	-MPZ mutations cause demyelinating or axonal neuropathies -AD or AR
CMT 3 (Dejerine-Sottas)	Multiple genes (*PMP22, EGR, MPZ*, periaxin)	-Severe -Very slow conduction
CMT type 2		-Axonal -Mainly AD
CMT 2a	*MFN2*	-20% of CMT2 -Mitochondrial dysfunction -Hearing loss
CMT 2b	*RAB7*	-Acromutilation -Mainly sensory
CMT X	Chromosome X, *GJB1* (gap-junction binding protein, also called connexin-32)	-Connexin mutations cause mixed demyelinating or axonal -Encephalopathy

Overall, the 5 most common forms of CMT are:
- CMT 1A (*PMP22* duplication)   37%
- CMT X (*GJB1/Cx32*)   10%
- HNPP (*PMP22* deletion)   6%
- CMT 1B (*MPZ*)   6%
- CMT 2A (*MFN*)   3%

Hereditary Neuropathy with Predisposition to Pressure Palsies (HNPP)

Caused by *PMP22* deletion, results in distal slowing, tomaculae on teased fiber preparation, and AD inheritance. De novo mutations are common. Can have brain white matter lesions seen on MRI.

Other Inherited Conditions that Cause Neuropathy

Condition	Gene/Protein/Enzyme	Unique Finding(s)
Amyloid polyneuropathy	-Transthyretin gene (*TTR*) -Can also be acquired	-Multiple neuropathic conditions: carpal tunnel syndrome, painful small fiber neuropathy, autonomic symptoms, CIDP-like -Cardiomyopathy -Hepatomegaly -Diagnosed with: fat pad biopsy, light chain elevation, or *hATTR* (transthyretin) genetic testing -Hereditary treated with RNA interference (patisiran) or antisense oligonucleotide (inotersen)
Fabry Disease	-X linked, so affects men more severely. Women can by symptomatic because of X-inactivation -*GLA* gene -Deficiency of lysosomal α-galactosidase A (α-GAL). Leads to progressive cellular accumulation of glycosphingolipids, particularly globotriaosylceramide (GL-3)	-Causes a painful neuropathy in the palms and soles, hypohydrosis, angiokeratomas in pelvic/inguinal/genital regions -Starts around age 20 -Worse with alcohol, stress, fever, hot weather -Results in renal failure, cardiac conditions, and stroke -Treated with enzyme replacement agalsidase beta
Tangier Disease	-Defect in *ABCA1* transporter -Rare and AR	-Polyneuropathy, proximal pseudo syrinx, patchy, facial diplegia -Elevated cholesterol -Orange tonsils
Refsum Disease	-*PHYH* gene mutation -Build-up of phytanic acid	-Starts in childhood/adolescence with night blindness -Demyelinating neuropathy -Deafness -Cardiomyopathy -Very high spinal fluid protein
Hexosaminidase A (Tay-Sachs)	-*HEXA* gene	-Cerebellar dysfunction with truncal ataxia, pyramidal signs, psychosis, and atrophy -Symmetric weakness -Low amplitude CMAPs and sensory nerve action potentials (SNAPs)
Porphyria	-Multiple different genes	-Axonal neuropathy -GI symptoms -Psychosis, hallucinations -More common in women, usually age 18-40 -Diagnosed through elevated urine porphobilinogens

Acquired Neuropathies

The most common cause of polyneuropathy, both in the United States and worldwide, is <u>diabetes</u>. The typical presentation is a distal, symmetric polyneuropathy that progresses over years. It typically has an axonal appearance by electrodiagnostic testing.

Rare manifestations of diabetes include diabetic amyotrophy, painless diabetic lumbosacral plexopathy, diabetic neuritis, and insulin neuritis. These processes likely have immune/vasculitic components.

Immune Mediated Processes

Condition	Antibodies	Unique Finding(s)
Guillain-Barre Syndrome	-GD1a – acute motor axonal neuropathy (AMAN) -GM1 – AMAN and multifocal motor neuropathy (MMN) -GM1b – AMAN -GQ1b – Miller-Fischer (95% of cases), triad of ataxia, areflexia, ophthalmoplegia -GT1a – pharyngeal-cervical-brachial	-Preceding gastroenteritis, upper respiratory infection, vaccination, or surgery -Treated with IVIG or plasmapheresis -Progresses over < 4 weeks
Sensory neuronopathy (sensory ganglionopathy)	-Anti Hu, CV2/CRMP antibodies -Can be seen in Sjogren's with SSA/SSB antibodies	-80% female -80% with pain -Other symptoms include limbic encephalitis, seizures, cerebellar ataxia, autonomic dysfunction (30%) -Can be from autoimmune, paraneoplastic, B6 deficiency -Testing: absent SNAPs, normal CMAPs, high spinal fluid protein
Chronic inflammatory demyelinating polyradiculoneuropathy (CIDP)	Distal acquired demyelinating symmetric (DADS) variant with anti-MAG antibody	-Progresses over > 8 weeks -Symmetric proximal and distal weakness -Multifocal acquired demyelinating sensory and motor (MADSAM) variant, also called Lewis-Sumner variant -IVIG and prednisone are first-line treatments -Rituximab for DADS variant

More Immune Mediated Processes

Multifocal motor neuropathy (MMN)	GM1	-More often in men, age 30-50. -Conduction block is usually present. -Arms more affected than legs. -Responds to IVIG (do not use prednisone)
Neuralgic amyotrophy (also called Parsonage-Turner Syndrome)	-Usually not hereditary -Hereditary form from Sept9 (chromosome 17) gene mutations. They have hypotelorism, narrow face, short stature, and syndactyly.	-Antecedent illness or surgery, severe shoulder pain for 2 weeks, replaced by dull ache -Weakness and atrophy develop. Motor nerves (suprascapular, long thoracic, musculocutaneous, anterior interosseous) involved -Ultrasound may show torsion and/or hourglass enlargement of radial, posterior interosseous, anterior interosseous, median, or ulnar nerves
Mononeuritis multiplex	-Polyarteritis nodosa – most common, associated with hepatitis B and C -Eosinophilic granulomatosis with polyangiitis (EGPA), also called "Churg-Strauss" – p ANCA antibody, asthma, eosinophilia -Granulomatosis with polyangiitis (GPA), formerly called "Wegener's" – c ANCA antibody, renal involvement	-Vasculitis causes mononeuritis multiplex, which is focal, patchy, and often painful
Paraproteinemias	-IgG lambda – POEMS, elevated VEGF -IgM – MAG demyelinating polyneuropathy, DADS phenotype, Waldenstrom, no conduction block -Kappa light chains – multiple myeloma -Monoclonal light chains – systemic amyloidosis	-10% of people over age 60 have non-specific M spikes (MGUS)

Motor Neuron Diseases (MND)

This is a broad category of diseases, which includes amyotrophic lateral sclerosis (ALS), spinal muscular atrophy (SMA), infectious motor neuron disease (polio, West Nile Virus), and hereditary spastic paraparesis.

MND Type	Chromosome/Gene/Protein	Unique Finding(s)
Amyotrophic lateral sclerosis (ALS)	-*C9ORF72* hexanucleotide repeat, associated with frontotemporal dementia, most common -*SOD1* second most common -20+ other known genes	-10% familial (AD) -Life expectancy 4 years -Riluzole – glutamate inhibitor -Edaravone – free radical scavenger
Bulbar-onset ALS		Life expectancy 2 years
Progressive muscular atrophy (PMA; an ALS variant)		-Lower motor neuron only -Life expectancy of 8 years
Primary lateral sclerosis (PLS; an ALS variant)		-Upper motor neuron only -Life expectancy of 15 years
Spinal muscular atrophy (SMA)	-*SMN1* gene (AR) on 5q chromosome -*SMN2* copy number determines disease severity (the more copies the less severe) -5q type is 95% of SMA	-See separate table -Proximal and symmetric -Scoliosis is common -Vulnerable to fasting -Treated with nusinersen (intrathecal antisense oligonucleotide) or IV *SMN1* gene replacement (Zolgensma)
Distal SMA	-Rare, 5% of SMA -Multiple genes (dynactin, *HSP 22*, *HSP 27*, glycyl-tRNA synthetase, and SMA with respiratory distress (*SMARD*))	
Spinal and bulbar muscular atrophy (SBMA, Kennedy's Disease)	-X-linked -Androgen receptor gene -CAG repeat	-Bulbar weakness -High CK -Sensory involvement on NCS -Gynecomastia -Slowly progressive, normal life-span
Infectious MND		-Polio -West Nile virus
Hereditary spastic paraparesis (HSP)	->20 genes identified -Usually AD	-Uncomplicated: only lower extremity spasticity -Complicated: may involve cognition, upper extremities, bladder, sensation, etc.

Spinal Muscular Atrophy
SMA has been categorized using different approaches over the years, with the 3 main systems being age of onset, best motor milestone attained, and SMN2 copy number.

SMA Type	SMN2 #	Onset	Motor Milestone	Prognosis	Eponym
0	0-1	Birth	Non-sitter	Death in utero	
1	1-2	0-6 months	Non-sitter	Death before age 2	Werdnig-Hoffmann
2	2-3	6-18 months	Sitter	Live at least 20 years	
3	2-4	> 18 months	Stander	Normal lifespan	Kugelberg-Welander
4	4+	Adult	Stander	Normal lifespan	

Differential Diagnoses for Bulbar-onset ALS
Spinal and bulbar muscular atrophy (Kennedy's Disease)
MuSK MG – African American females, tongue atrophy can occur
Oculopharyngeal muscular dystrophy – abnormal eye movements, AD, *PAPBN1* gene GCG repeat, French-Canadian ancestry
Pharyngeal-cervico-brachial variant of GBS – GT1a antibodies, acute onset
Brainstem process – tumor, stroke, multiple sclerosis
Cerebellar process – spinocerebellar ataxia
Transthyretin Familial Amyloid Polyneuropathy (TTR-FAP) – AD, amyloidosis more often causes macroglossia (especially in light-chain amyloidosis) but can cause tongue atrophy and fasciculations; severe polyneuropathy, dysautonomia, and dementia can occur

Differential Diagnoses for Myeloneuropathies (spinal cord and polyneuropathy)
B12 deficiency
Nitrous oxide toxicity – similar to B12 deficiency, although more acute, can exacerbate B12 deficiency
Copper deficiency – pancytopenia, from zinc excess, sometimes from denture cream
Vitamin E deficiency
Adrenomyeloneuropathy (x-linked) – typical brain changes of myelin on MRI, elevated very long chain fatty acids, peroxisomal disease, *ABCD* gene mutation
Metachromatic leukodystrophy
Pelizaeus-Merzbacher (x-linked) – spastic paraplegia
Adult polyglucosan body disease – incontinence, dementia, and neuropathy
Tay-Sachs (hexosaminidase A deficiency) – symmetric weakness, can have cerebellar signs
Cerebrotendinous xanthomatosis – AR, tendon xanthomas, cataracts, chronic diarrhea, dementia, ataxia
Allgrove Syndrome – Triple A syndrome - alacrima, achalasia, adrenal insufficiency. They can have a sensorimotor syndrome

HIV – elevated white cell count in spinal fluid
HTLV I/II – tropical paraparesis

Other Conditions

Malignant Nerve Sheath Tumors
50% from neurofibromatosis type 1
10% from previous radiation

Obstetric Brachial Plexopathies
Common: Erb's palsy (C5-6). Shoulder adduction, internal rotation, pronation of forearm ("waiter's tip" position).
Uncommon: Klumpke's (C8). Hand paralysis and Horner's syndrome.

Radiculopathies
Weakness
Genitourinary dysfunction
Intractable pain for more than 6 weeks

Lumbar extension make stenosis worse
Should abduction helps cervical radiculopathy

Radiation Plexitis
Starts months to years after treatment, can even occur multiple decades after treatment
Slowly progressive
Painless
Myokymia may be present on EMG, but not in all muscles
Upper brachial plexus, lumbosacral plexus
Commonly from treatment of breast and lung cancer with high doses of radiation

Differential for Flaccid Paralysis with Spinal Fluid Pleocytosis

HIV
CMV
West Nile Virus
Sarcoidosis
Lyme

Treatment of Neuropathic Pain

Pregabalin and gabapentin – calcium channels
Capsaicin – substance p
Topical lidocaine – blocks sodium channels
Antidepressants – norepinephrine reuptake inhibition

Scapular Winging

3 main muscles stabilize the scapula – the trapezius (CN XI, spinal accessory), rhomboids (C5, upper trunk, dorsal scapular), and serratus anterior (C5-7, long thoracic)

Trapezius weakness (spinal accessory nerve) – scapula is more lateral than usual, inferior angle rotates medially (like with serratus anterior weakness), worse with arm abduction and external rotation

Rhomboid weakness (dorsal scapular) – scapula is more lateral than usual including the inferior angle, worse with slow forward arm raise

Serratus anterior weakness (long thoracic nerve) – scapula is more medial than usual, inferior angle rotates medially, winging of the medial border of the scapula, lateral shoulder appears lower, worse with arm extended forward and raised (forward flexion)

Chapter 4. GENERAL NEUROMUSCULAR TOPICS

Toxic Neuromuscular Conditions

Drug/Toxin	Neuromuscular Finding(s)	Other Finding(s)
Cisplatin	Sensory ganglionopathy Continue toxicity after stopping (coasting)	Polyneuropathy
Thallium	Scalp hair loss	-Axonal neuropathy -GI symptoms -GBS mimic -Ataxia -Encephalopathy/coma
Lead	Wrist and finger drop	-Similar to porphyria -Axonal neuropathy -GI symptoms -Microcytic anemia -Renal failure -Gout
Gold	Isolated polyneuropathy	
Arsenic	Polyneuropathy	Mees' lines (changes in nailbed)
Mercury	CNS symptoms	-Axonal neuropathy -Postural tremor
Zinc	-Copper deficiency -Myeloneuropathy -Pancytopenia	
Glue (n-hexane) Hexacarbons	-Myeloneuropathy -Giant axons filled with filaments	-Some demyelination -Conduction block
TNF alpha Infliximab Adalimumab Etanercept Tacrolimus	-Demyelinating neuropathy -EDX like CIDP	
Amiodarone	Neuromyopathy with chronic use	
Colchicine	Neuromyopathy	
Chloroquine	Neuromyopathy	Authophagic vacuoles
Dapsone	Distal motor neuropathy	
Zidovudine	Myopathy	
Organophosphates	-Salivation, lacrimation, urination, defecation, emesis (SLUDE) (muscarinic) -Weakness and fasciculations (nicotinic) -Delayed polyneuropathy	

More Toxic Neuromuscular Conditions

Cyclosporine	Myopathy with type 2 atrophy	
Steroids	Myopathy with type 2 atrophy	No fibs or positive waves
Pyridoxine (B6)	-Sensory ganglionopathy -Seizures -Dermatitis	High or low causes toxicity
Vitamin D	-Myalgias -Myopathy	
Vitamin E	-Dorsal column dysfunction -Myopathy	
Thiamine	-Polyneuropathy (dry beriberi) -Confabulation	

Trinucleotide Repeat Disorders

Spinocerebellar ataxias
Friedreich's ataxia – GAA repeat in frataxin (*FXN*) gene
Oculopharnygeal muscular dystrophy (OPMD) - CGC
Fascioscapulohumeral dystrophy (FSHD) – fewer number of repeats
Myotonic dystrophy – CTG, chromosome 19
Spinal and bulbar muscular atrophy (Kennedy's Disease) - CAG

Diseases That Improve with Exercise

LEMS
Myotonia congenita
McArdle's Disease – second wind phenomenon

Genes with Multiple Phenotypes

Dysferlin – LGMDR 2, distal myopathy, hyperCKemia
Fukutin – LGMD 2I (common, cardiomyopathy), congenital muscular dystrophy
LMNA A/C – Emery-Dreifuss muscular dystrophy, congenital muscular dystrophy with rigid spine, cardiomyopathy, AR axonal CMT
Myelin protein zero (MPZ) – AD and AR, demyelinating and axonal polyneuropathy, Dejerine-Sottas

Ataxias

In those diagnosed under age 30, > 75% are from Friedreich's. This is an AR inherited disease caused by a GAA repeat in the FXN gene which results in decreased expression of the mitochondrial protein frataxin. It is associated with scoliosis, heart disease (90%), diabetes (10%), hearing loss, and vision loss.

Spinocerebellar ataxias have AD inheritance.

Scoliosis

Dextroscoliosis – the spine curves to the right, often thoracic, and often from neuromuscular causes
Levoscoliosis – the spine curves to the left, often lumbar, and often idiopathic

Chapter 5. CLINICAL NEUROPHYSIOLOGY

Action Potentials

Depolarization   Sodium rushes in
Repolarization   Increased potassium ion permeability
Refractory period   3 milliseconds duration

Nerve Conduction Studies

The cathode (black) is the negative electrode and positioned distal to the anode during stimulation for routine nerve conduction studies. One way to remember this is if the stimulator electrodes are accidently reversed, the anode is distal and it causes "anodal block" artifact of the stimulating impulse. The recording electrode is also black (black-to-black is the standard set up). The reference electrode is 3-4 cm from the active/recording electrode.

Ohm's law: Current (I) = Voltage (V)/Resistance (R)

Filters (mainly affect waveform shape – duration and amplitude)

CMAP: made of more low frequency potentials
SNAP: made of more high frequency potentials

Excess low frequencies cause baseline wandering and increased duration. Excess high frequencies obscure small waveforms.

Low frequency (high-pass) filter (adjustments mainly affect duration):
 Increase the filter: fewer waveforms, decreases amplitude, decreases duration
 Decrease the filter: more waveforms, increases amplitude, increases duration

High frequency (low-pass) filter (adjustments mainly affect amplitude):
 Increase the filter: more waveforms, increases the amplitude, decreases duration (accentuates high frequency waveforms)
 Decrease the filter: fewer waveforms, decreases the amplitude, increases duration (accentuates low frequency waveforms)

Technical Artifacts

Artifact	Finding
Submaximal stimulation	Low amplitudes
Anode block	Stimulator is reversed, low amplitude
Virtual cathode	Excessive stimulation, latency is decreased
Close electrodes	Positioning the active (recording) and reference electrodes too close decreases the amplitude because of rejection of waveforms that are recorded by both electrodes at the same time
Cool limb	Long latency, slow velocity, increased sensory amplitude, improve neuromuscular junction transmission, more prominent in sensory compared to motor studies

EMG Findings
Types of Spontaneous EMG Activity

Discharge	Generator	Description	Frequency
End plate noise	End plate	Seashell, from miniature end-plate potentials	
End plate spikes	Muscle fiber	Random, like popping grease, from nerve twig potentials	50-100 Hz
Fibrillations	Muscle fiber	Regular, rain on tin roof, decreased by hypoxic states	0.5-15 Hz
Positive sharp wave	Muscle fiber	Regular, thud	
Complex repetitive discharge	Muscle fiber	Mechanical like motor boat, from ephaptic fiber transmission	
Myotonic discharge	Muscle fiber	Dive bomber, waxing and waning	20-100 Hz
Fasciculation	Motor unit	Random, pops	
Doublet/triplet	Motor unit	Random, groups of motor units or fasciculations, worse with hyperventilation and hypoglycemia, different meaning if spontaneous vs voluntary	
Myokymia	Motor unit	Marching soldiers	2-60 Hz
Neuromyotonia	Motor unit	Very fast, ping with waning	100-300 Hz
Cramp	Motor unit	Irregular at termination	40-150 Hz

Causes of Myotonia (dive bomber, waxing and waning, 20-100 Hz)

Clinical myotonia AND EMG myotonia
- Myotonic dystrophy 1 and 2
- Schwartz-Jampel (chondrodystrophic myotonia)
- Myotonia congenita (*CLCN1* gene)

Clinical paramyotonia AND EMG myotonia
- Paramyotonia congenital – exercise makes it worse and it worsens with cold
- Hyperkalemic periodic paralyses (*SCN4* gene)

No clinical myotonia AND EMG myotonia
- Pompe Disease (acid maltase or acid alpha glucosidase deficiency, GSD II)
- Polymyositis

Causes of Neuromyotonia (ping with amplitude change, 100-300 Hz)

- Isaacs's Syndrome (acquired, paraneoplastic, hereditary) – voltage-gated potassium channel antibodies, CMAP after-discharges
- Morvan Syndrome (rare, autoimmune, usually resolves, neuromyotonia, cramps, delirium, insomnia)

Causes of Myokymia (marching soldiers, 2-60 Hz)

Radiation plexitis
Brainstem glioma
Multiple sclerosis (facial)
Chronic demyelinating focal lesion, such as with carpal tunnel syndrome

Sequence of Changes Following Complete Nerve Transection

3 days	Loss of CMAP
7 days	Loss of SNAP
14 days	Development of fibs and positive sharp waves
30 days	Collateral sprouting, which results in larger voluntary motor units

Nerve Conduction Study Findings

Causes of Repetitive Stimulation Decrement at 3 Hz stimulation
Myasthenia gravis
Lambert-Eaton myasthenia syndrome
ALS
Myotonic disorders
Centronuclear myopathy

Causes of CMAP after-discharges
Non-dystrophic myotonias (myotonia congenita and paramyotonia congenita)
Acetylcholinesterase deficiency congenital myasthenic syndrome
Slow channel congenital myasthenic syndrome
Organophosphate toxicity
Isaac's syndrome
Envenomation with potassium channel poisons

Exercise Tests
Short (exercise for 10 seconds)
    Myotonia congenita – CMAP drops then improves
    Paramyotonia congenita – CMAP drops and stays down

Long (exercise intermittently for 5 minutes)
    HypoKPP – slowly drops over 60 minutes

Autonomic testing
QSART is abnormal with peripheral cause and normal with central causes.

Ross syndrome is asymmetric, focal autonomic neuropathy (Adie pupil)

Neuromuscular Ultrasound

Carpal tunnel syndrome results in the following median nerve changes: increased cross-sectional area, increased vascularity with Doppler, decreased echogenicity, and decreased mobility.

Fibular mononeuropathy: an intraneural ganglion cyst occurs in ~20% of those with a foot drop and no clear etiology (such as weight loss, immobilization, and habitual leg crossing). Proper surgical intervention is required.

CMT vs CIDP: in general CMT results in diffuse, symmetric nerve enlargement, whereas CIDP results in multifocal nerve enlargement (often affecting the brachial plexus).

Idiopathic brachial plexitis (Parsonage-Turner syndrome): the pathology is not actually in the brachial plexus (it's a misnomer). Focal sausage-like enlargement, with nerve fascicle twisting, can be seen in the radial and median nerves in the arm.

Inflammatory myopathy: early on the muscle may be swollen with increased Doppler signal, but as the disease progresses the muscle may become atrophic and hyperechoic.

Differential for Acquired Demyelinating Polyneuropathy

Guillain-Barre Syndrome – weakness over 4 weeks, autonomic instability, facial and respiratory weakness
CIDP – less likely than Guillain-Barre to affect cranial nerves
Immunomodulatory medications
Monoclonal gammopathies
Autoimmune diseases – lupus, Sjogren's, Crohn's, ulcerative colitis
Porphyria
Heavy metal toxicity
Refsum Disease

Key Muscles for Differentiating Innervation

Pronator teres (median and C6-7 innervated) – C7 radiculopathy vs radial mononeuropathy
Short head of the biceps femoris (only fibular innervated muscle above the knee) – common vs deep fibular mononeuropathy
Tibialis posterior/gluteus medius – L5 radiculopathy vs fibular mononeuropathy, both are L5 but not fibular innervated
Adductor longus – L3 radiculopathy vs femoral mononeuropathy, the adductor longus is innervated by the obturator nerve

Thenar Muscles

1. Abductor pollicis brevis (median nerve)
2. Opponens pollicis (median nerve)
3. Flexor pollicis brevis, superficial head (median nerve)
4. Flexor pollicis brevis, deep head (ulnar nerve)

The adductor pollicis is near the thenar muscles (just distal and deep) and is innervated by the ulnar nerve.

The sartorius is the only muscle to flex the hip and knee.

www.ingramcontent.com/pod-product-compliance
Lightning Source LLC
Chambersburg PA
CBHW080437220526
45465CB00009B/3322